MEDICINE BALL TRAINING

*A Complete Book of Medicine Ball
Exercises for Coaches of All Sports*

By
Zoltan Tenke
Andy Higgins

Illustrations By
Eric Little

SPORT BOOKS PUBLISHER 1992

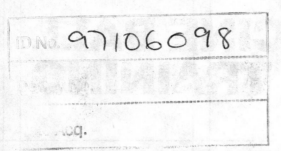

Canadian Cataloguing in Publication Data

Tenke, Zoltan.
  Medicine ball training

ISBN 0-920905-40-4

1. Medicine ball. 2. Callisthenics. I. Higgins, Andy.
II. Title.

GV496.T47 1992   613.7'13 C92-095260-7

Distribution worldwide by
Sport Books Publisher
278 Robert Street
Toronto, Ontario M5S 2K8
Canada

Printed in the United States

CONTENTS

FOREWORD

Numerous articles and texts have been written on the technical aspects of almost every sport. An equal number of directions are available on how to plan ideal training programs. Frequently, however, writers have neglected to supply a sufficient amount of supporting resource information to assist coaches in the development of a basic and varied training program.

What follows is a selection of medicine ball exercises that may be used in developing either the general fitness and condition of the athlete or the more specific components of any athletic endeavour.

For the most part, the exercises are performed in pairs. This allows for efficient use of practice time as well as for group interaction so important in any sport, and especially in those that are inherently individual.

This book will definitely be an extremely useful addition to the resource materials of any coach in any sport.

Authors

INTRODUCTION

The medicine ball is again becoming a very popular, useful, and enjoyable piece of light equipment. An old expression in Europe says "He who uses the medicine ball does not need medicine!" Undoubtedly, these exercises are very good medicine for athletes.

The medicine ball is among the most versatile pieces of equipment that may be used in athletic preparation. There are exercises suited for training all the muscles of the body, and the repertoire of exercises is not only large but extremely varied. It is possible to perform mobility exercises, strength developing exercises, throwing exercises, as well as games, relays, and competitions, all of which have a beneficial effect on general fitness.

The mobility exercises are used in the general warm-up, but because of the weight of the ball they are more intense than the callisthenic exercises. In fact, all mobility exercises, because of the weight of the ball, are also strengthening exercises.

The strength developing medicine ball exercises may be dynamic (isotonic),static (isometric), or a combination of both.

The mobility and strength developing exercises may be used to develop isolated muscle groups, and by employing a correct selection of exercises, all the muscles of the body may be involved.

The many single and double throw exercises that involve the entire body are especially good for developing smooth, co-ordinated movement. These exercises are appropriate for developing total fitness.

The medicine ball (as any other ball) may be used effectively in games, relays, and competitions.

It is obvious that the medicine ball has a variety of uses in preparing athletes and developing general fitness in people of all ages and abilities (from children to high performance athletes), and may be used in innovative and challenging ways to accomplish these ends.

It is important to consider the age and the stage of development of the individual involved when selecting the medicine ball. Ideally, it should range from 1/2 kg (1 lb) to 5kg (12 lb).

For warm-up and preparation exercises or strength developing exercises, it is best to have the group in a straight line or in rows spaced about two metres apart. With small groups, a circle or a semi-circle is a good formation.

The throws are best done in pairs in two open lines facing each other. The distance between the partners will depend upon the age, the level of development, and the difficulty of the throws.

Standing throws should be taught at the beginning. Later, individuals may be introduced to throws from a kneeling position, and finally from a lying position.

To avoid finger injuries from the weight of the ball it is important to learn the proper catching technique. It is most effective to receive the incoming ball in the angle of the arm at the elbow and to use the other hand to cover the ball and prevent it from spinning away.

DIRECTIONS FOR USING THIS BOOK

This book consists of four categories of exercises:

1. General warm-up and preparation exercises.
2. Strength developing exercises.
3. Throwing exercises.
4. Competitions, relays, and games.

The coach will see that there are a variety of ways to use these exercise categories. In fact, s/he may use exercises from all categories in one session. However, this should be done only in the preparation period of the year, and in this case, the entire session consist of medicine ball exercises.

During the remaining training periods of the year, exercises from only one or two categories should be used to complement or supplement the other aspects of a particular session. For example: selected exercises from *one* of the above categories or combinations, such as a) general warm up and strength developing exercises, or b) general warm up and throwing exercises, or c) strength developing and throwing exercises, etc.

At times other than during the preparation period of the year it is unwise to load a session heavily with medicine ball exercises.

In general preparation it is essential to select a number of different exercises from each category to ensure that all the muscle groups are involved. For this reason, each category has a number of groups of exercises and each group has many samples.

In addition, the exercises within each group are graded in terms of difficulty.

With only a minimum of time for planning it is possible for the coach to select exercises from each group to meet whatever his or her needs may be. The session may be very specific or it may be extremely general. With respect to the latter, there are enough exercises to ensure that the entire body is properly involved.

Because of the large number of possibilities for combinations of exercises and exercise variations, it is relatively simple to create training sessions that are continually challenging, different enough to be interesting, and effective enough to guarantee continual fitness improvement.

1.1 HOPPING EXERCISES

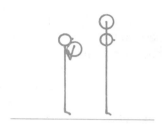

E1 **With the ball held at the chest.**
Hopping 3 times on the spot (1-3) and
on (4) the ball is extended overhead
to the high position.

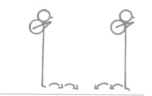

E2 **With the ball at the back
of the neck.**
Double leg hopping forwards 4 times
(1-4) and 4 times double leg hopping
backwards (5-8).

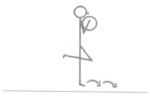

E3 **With the ball at the chest.**
Hopping forwards 4 times on left leg
(1-4) and then the right leg (5-8).

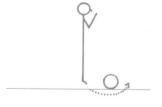

E4 **With the ball on the ground and
standing behind the ball in basic
erect stance.**
Hopping around the ball to the left
and then to the right.

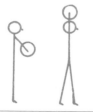

E5 **With the ball in deep position.**
Hopping 3 times on spot (1-3) and on
(4), jump to straddle with ball in high
position.

E6 With the ball on the ground and standing to the right of the ball.
Hopping 3 times on the spot (1-3) and on (4) hop over ball to left side. Repeat.

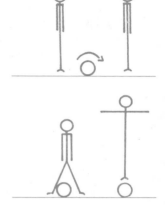

E7 Straddle stance over the ball.
Hopping in straddle position 3 times (1-3) and hop high above the ball and close legs while in the air (4). Repeat.

E8 Basic erect stance behind the ball.
Hopping on the spot 3 times (1-3). Jump over the ball with 180° left or right turn (4).

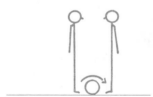

E9 With the ball in deep position.
Hopping 3 times on the spot (1-3) and on (4) jump to straddle with ball at shoulder level.

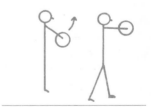

E10 Basic erect stance behind the ball.
Hopping on the spot 3 times (1-3), jump over the ball (4), hopping 3 times on spot (5-7), jump over the ball backwards (8).

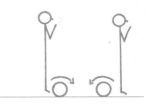

1.2 ARM EXERCISES

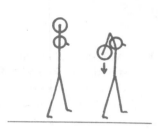

E1 **Straddle stance with ball in high position.**
Bend arms backwards and press down 3 times behind neck (1-3), extend arms to start (4).

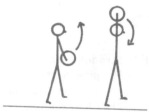

E2 **Straddle stance with ball in deep position.**
Swing ball to high position (1) and return to deep position (2).

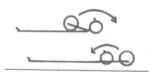

E3 **Lying back with ball in deep position.**
Swing ball to high position (1) and return to deep position (2).

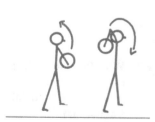

E4 **Straddle stance with ball in deep position.**
Swing ball to high position and bend arms backwards (1) then swing with extension through high position to starting position (2).

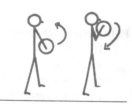

E5 **Straddle stance with ball in deep position.**
Swing ball in an arc to chest (1) and again in an arc to deep position (2).

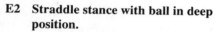

E6 **Straddle with ball in deep position behind the body.**
Swing the ball upwards 3 times (1-3) and return to start (4).

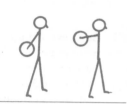

E7 **Straddle stance with ball in deep position.**
Swing ball to shoulder position (1), swing ball to deep position (2), swing ball to high position (3), swing ball to deep position (4).

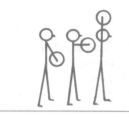

E8 **Straddle stance with ball in high position.**
Swing ball down and to the left side backwards (1). Return to start (2). Repeat to the right.

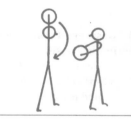

E9 **Straddle stance with ball in high position.**
Circling to left twice (1-2) and twice to the right (3-4).

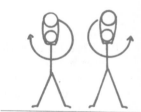

E10 **Lying back in straddle position with ball in high position.**
Swing ball forward to left side of body (1), return to start (2). Repeat to right side.

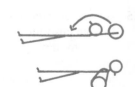

1.3 LEG EXERCISES

**E1 Basic erect stance with ball
in forward position.**
Lower to supported squat position
and bounce 3 times (1-3) and return
to starting position (4).

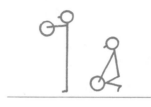

**E2 Basic erect stance with ball
on top of head.**
Lower to squat position and bounce
3 times (1-3). Return to starting
position (4).

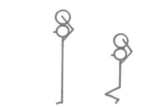

**E3 Basic erect stance with ball
in high position.**
Lower to squat position and bounce
3 times (1-3) while lowering ball
behind neck. Return to starting
position (4).

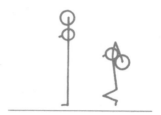

**E4 Basic erect stance with ball
in deep position.**
Lower to squat position and raise the
ball to forward position (1-2). Return
to starting position (3-4).

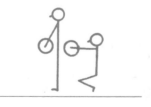

**E5 Basic erect stance with ball
in high position.**
Lower to squat position and bring
ball to forward position. Bounce 3
times (1-3) and return to starting
position (4).

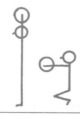

**E6   Basic erect stance with ball
in deep position.**
With ball behind the back lower to
squat position and bounce 3 times
(1-3). Return to starting position (4).

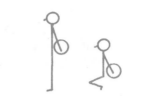

**E7   Basic erect stance with ball
behind neck.**
Step forward to lunge position and
bounce 3 times (1-3). Return to
starting position (4). Repeat with
opposite leg.

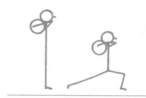

**E8   Deep straddle stance with ball
in high position.**
Shift weight to left leg, lower ball to
chest and bounce 3 times (1-3).
Return to starting position (4). Repeat
to opposite side.

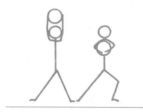

**E9   Basic erect stance with ball
in deep position.**
Step forward to lunge position swing
ball to high position and bounce 3
times (1-3). Return to starting
position (4). Repeat with opposite
leg.

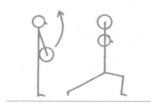

**E10 Basic erect stance with ball
at the chest.**
Lower to squat and raise ball to high
position, bounce 3 times (1-3). Return
to starting position (4).

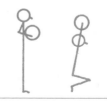

1.4 LEG SWINGING

**E1   Lying back position, with knees bent
and ball in front shoulder position.**
Swing left leg to touch ball (1). Return
to starting position (2). Repeat with
right leg.

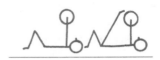

**E2   Basic erect stance with ball in front
shoulder position.**
Swing left leg to touch ball (1).
Return to starting position (2). Repeat
with right leg.

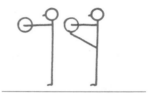

**E3   Basic erect stance with ball in high
diagonal position.**
Swing left leg to touch ball (1).
Return to starting position (2) and
repeat with right leg (3-4).

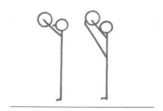

**E4   Lying back with ball in high
diagonal position.**
Swing left leg to touch ball (1).
Return to starting position (2). Repeat
with right leg.

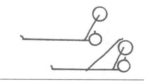

**E5   Prone lying position, ball
in high position.**
Swing left leg backwards (1). Return
to staring position (2). Repeat with
right leg.

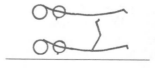

**E6 Basic erect stance with ball
in high position.**
Swing left leg forwards and lower
ball to meet in front shoulder position
(1). Return to starting position (2).
Repeat with right leg.

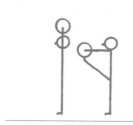

**E7 Basic erect stance with ball
in deep position.**
Swing left leg backwards with ball
swinging to high position (1). Return
to starting position (2). Repeat with
right leg.

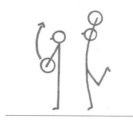

**E8 Basic sitting position with ball
in high position.**
Swing left leg forwards and ball
down to meet in high diagonal
position (1). Return to starting
position (2). Repeat with right leg.

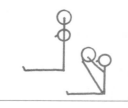

**E9 Basic erect stance with ball
in high position.**
Swing left leg sideways and ball
downwards and to left to meet (1).
Return to starting position (2). Repeat
with right leg.

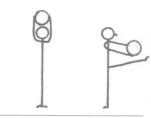

**E10 Narrow straddle stance with ball
in high position.**
Swing left leg to the right and swing
the ball to left shoulder position.

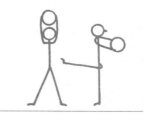

1.5 TRUNK BENDING FORWARD

**E1   Straddle stance behind the ball
with hands on top of ball.**
Bending forward with forehead
touching the ball (1), return
to start (2).

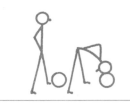

**E2   Straddle stance with ball in high
position.**
Trunk bending forward with ball
touching the ground (1), return
to start (2).

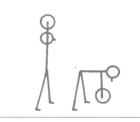

**E3   Straddle stance with ball
in high position.**
Trunk bending forward to left and
touch ball to ground outside of left
foot (1), return to start (2). Repeat to
right.

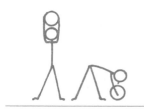

**E4   Straddle stance with ball in high
position.**
Trunk bending forward and swing
ball between legs 3 times (1-3), return
to start (4).

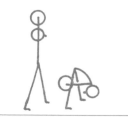

**E5   Straddle stance with ball in high
position.**
Trunk bending forward and swing
ball between legs to touch the
ground behind 3 times (1-3),
return to start (4).

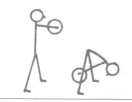

E6 **Seated in straddle position with ball on neck.**
Trunk bending forward 3 times (1-3) and return to start (4).

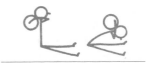

E7 **Erect stance with ball in high position.**
Bend trunk forward and swing ball down and backwards to left side with knee bouncing (1). With knee bouncing, swing ball to start (2), repeat to right side (3-4).

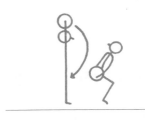

E8 **Straddle stance with ball in high position.**
Trunk bending forward 3 times: touch ball to ground outside of left foot (1), in front of body (2), outside of right foot (3), and swing back to starting position (4). Repeat to other side.

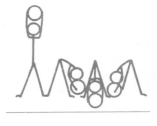

E9 **Seated in straddle position with ball in high position.**
Bend trunk forward, touching ball to ground (1). Return to start (2).

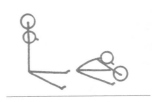

E10 **Straddle stance with ball behind the body in deep position.**
Trunk bending forward, swing ball upwards 3 times (1-3). Return to start (4).

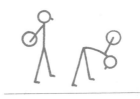

1.6 TRUNK BENDING BACKWARD

E1 **Straddle stance, ball behind the neck.**
Bend trunk backwards 3 times (1-3).
Return to starting position (4).

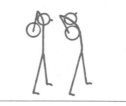

E2 **Straddle stance, ball on top of head.**
Bend trunk backwards 3 times (1-3).
Return to starting position (4).

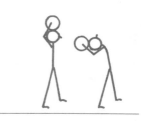

E3 **Straddle stance, ball in high position.**
Bend trunk backwards 3 times,
lowering ball to top of head (1-3).
Return to starting position (4).

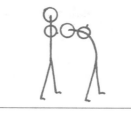

E4 **Straddle stance, ball in high position.**
Bend trunk backwards 3 times,
lowering back to neck position (1-3).
Return to starting position (4).

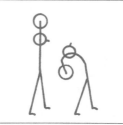

E5 **Straddle stance, ball in deep position behind the body.**
Bend trunk backwards 3 times (1-3).
Return to starting position (4).

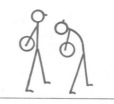

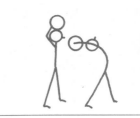

E6   Straddle stance, ball on top of head.
Bend the trunk backwards 3 times
extending ball to high position (1-3).
Return to starting position (4).

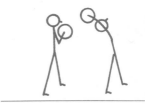

**E7   Straddle stance, ball
in front of chest.**
Bend trunk backwards 3 times raising
ball to high position (1-3). Return to
starting position (4).

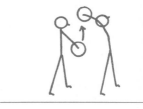

**E8   Straddle stance, ball
in deep position.**
Bend trunk backwards 3 times raising
ball to high position (1-3). Return to
starting position (4).

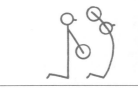

**E9   Straddle kneeling position
with ball in deep position.**
Bend trunk backwards 3 times
swinging ball to high position (1-3).
Return to starting position (4).

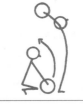

**E10 Supported squat position
with hands on ball.**
With knee extension swing ball to
high position with trunk bending
backwards 3 times (1-3). Return to
starting position (4).

1.7 TRUNK BENDING LATERALLY

E1 **Straddle stance with ball
     behind the neck.**
     Bend trunk to left 3 times (1-3).
     Return to starting position (4).
     Repeat to right side.

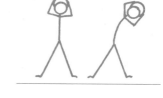

E2 **Straddle stance with ball
     on top of head.**
     Bend trunk to left 3 times (1-3).
     Return to starting position (4).
     Repeat to right side.

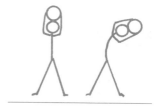

E3 **Straddle stance with ball
     in high position.**
     Bend trunk to left 3 times (1-3),
     lowering ball to top of head. Return
     to starting position (4). Repeat to
     right side.

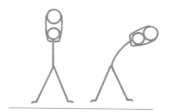

E4 **Straddle kneeling position,
     ball on top of head.**
     Bend trunk to left 3 times (1-3).
     Return to starting position (4).
     Repeat to right side.

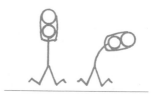

E5 **Straddle stance with ball on chest.**
     Bend trunk to left, raising ball to high
     position 3 times (1-3). Return to
     starting position (4). Repeat to right
     side.

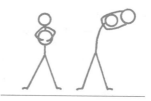

**E6 Straddle stance, ball
in high position.**
Bend trunk to left 3 times (1-3).
Return to starting position (4).
Repeat to right side.

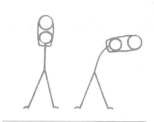

**E7 Straddle stance, ball
in high position.**
Circle ball 2 times (1-2) to the left,
bend trunk to the left 2 times (3-4).
Repeat to the right side.

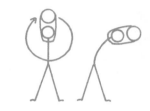

**E8 Wide straddle stance, ball
in high position.**
With right knee bouncing and trunk
bending left, lower ball to top of head
3 times (1-3). Return to starting
position (4). Repeat to left knee.

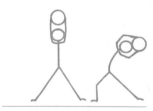

**E9 Straddle stance with arms in side
shoulder position and ball on left
palm.**
Bend trunk to the left 2 times (1-2), bend
trunk to right (3), swing left arm back to
starting position (4). (Ball remains on
right palm.) Repeat to other side.

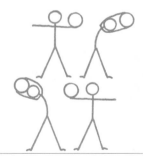

**E10 Wide straddle stance with ball on
top of head.**
Right knee bouncing and trunk
bending to left, raise ball to high
position 3 times (1-3). Return to
starting position (4). Repeat to other
side.

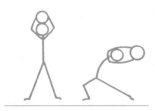

1.8 TRUNK TWISTING

E1 **Straddle stance with ball
in deep position.**
Twist the trunk to the left with ball
swinging to left shoulder position 3
times (1-3). Return to starting position
(4). Repeat to other side.

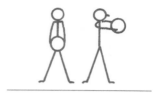

E2 **Kneeling straddle position
with ball in deep position.**
Twist the trunk to the left with ball
swinging to left shoulder position 3
times (1-3). Return to starting
position (4). Repeat to other side.

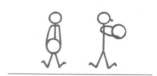

E3 **Straddle sitting position with ball
in deep position on floor.**
Twist the trunk to the left with ball
swinging to left shoulder position 3
times (1-3). Return to starting
position (4). Repeat to other side.

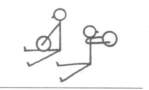

E4 **Lying back straddle position with
ball in front shoulder position.**
Lower the ball to the left on the floor
(1). Return to starting position (2).
Repeat to other side.

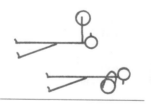

E5 **Straddle stance with ball
in left shoulder position.**
Swing ball horizontally to the right,
simultaneously twisting the trunk to
the right also (1). Return to starting
position (2). Repeat to the other side.

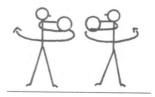

**E6 Kneeling position with ball
in front shoulder position.**
Step forward with the left leg, swing
ball to left shoulder position and twist
trunk 3 times to the left
(1-3). Return to starting position (4).
Repeat to other side.

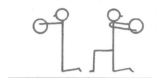

**E7 In pairs. Standing back to back about
1-2 metres apart and ball in front
shoulder position.**
Turn trunk and swing ball to left to begin
continuous passing of ball around from
one to other. Repeat to right side. This
exercise may also be performed by passing ball around in a figure eight pattern.

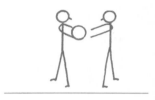

**E8 Straddle stance, ball
in deep position.**
With knee bouncing, swing ball to
left shoulder position and turn trunk
to left 2 times (1-2). Repeat to right
side.

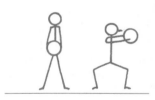

**E9 Straddle stance,
ball in high position.**
Swing ball in an arc down to left of
body in large figure eight pattern
(1-2). Repeat in other direction.

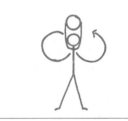

**E10 Basic erect stance, ball
in high position.**
Step forward to left lunge position,
swing ball to left shoulder position
and twist trunk to left 3 times (1-3).
Return to starting position (4). Repeat
to other side.

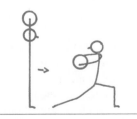

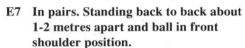

1.9 COMBINED TRUNK EXERCISES

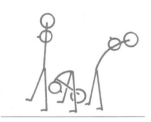

E1 **Straddle stance, ball in high position.**
Bend trunk forward and swing ball
between legs with trunk bouncing 2
times (1-2). Swing back to high
position and press trunk backwards 2
times (3-4).

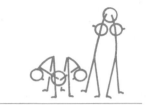

E2 **In pairs. Back to back,**
straddle position.
Move the ball in a circle by passing
between the legs and over the head.

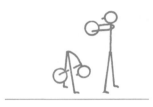

E3 **Straddle stance, ball in deep position.**
Bend the trunk forward with ball
swinging between the legs backwards 2
times (1-2). Return to erect position,
swing ball to left shoulder position and
rotate trunk to the left 2 times (3-4).
Return ball to low position (5). Repeat
to right side.

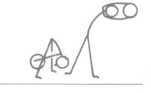

E4 **Straddle stance, ball in deep position.**
Bend the trunk forward with ball
swinging between the legs backwards 2
times (1-2). Swing ball to high position
and bend trunk to the left 2 times (3-4).
Return to start (5). Repeat to right side.

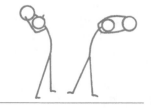

E5 **Straddle stance with ball**
on top of head.
Press the trunk backwards 2 times (1-
2), bend to the left while raising ball
to high position 2 times (3-4).

**E6 Straddle stance with ball
in left shoulder position.**
Swing ball horizontally with trunk
turning 4 times (1-4), then in trunk
bent forward position repeat exercise
4 times (5-8) in vertical plane.

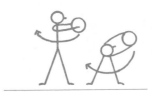

**E7 Straddle stance with flat back and
trunk in horizontal position, ball
on neck.**
Circle the trunk to the left 4 times (1-4)
and opposite direction 4 times (5-8).

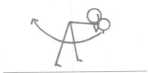

**E8 Straddle stance with ball in left
shoulder position.**
Swing ball horizontally with trunk
turning 4 times (1-4). Repeat 4 times
(5-8) with knee bouncing on each
swing (1/4 squat only).

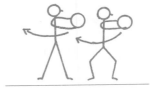

**E9 Straddle stance with flat back and
trunk in horizontal position, ball on
top of head.**
Circle the trunk to the left 4 times
(1-4) and then repeat to the right side
(5-8).

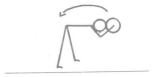

**E10 Straddle stance with flat back and
trunk in horizontal position, ball
in high position.**
Circle the trunk to the left 4 times
(1-4) and then repeat to the right
side (5-8).

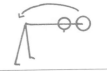

2.1 ARMS AND SHOULDERS

E1 **Straddle stance with ball in forward position.**
Moving the ball to the left, pass it around the trunk from one hand to the other 4 times (1-4). Repeat in the other direction.

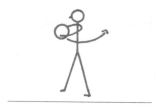

E2 **Straddle stance with ball at the chest.**
Press ball to forward position (1) hold for 2 counts (2-3). Return to chest (4).

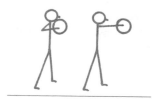

E3 **Straddle stance with ball in high position.**
Lower ball to left shoulder (1), return to high position (2), lower to right shoulder (3). Return to starting position (4).

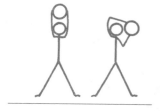

E4 **Straddle stance with ball in deep position.**
Raise ball to high diagonal (1), hold for 2 counts (2-3). Lower to starting position (4).

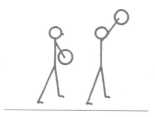

E5 **Lying in straddle supine position with ball on chest.**
Press ball to high diagonal position (1), hold for 2 counts (2-3). Return to starting position (4).

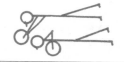

**E6   Straddle stance with ball
     in forward position.**
Raise to high position (1) and
lower to starting position (2).

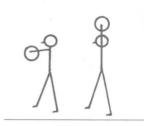

**E7   Straddle stance with ball
     in deep position.**
Swing the ball to high position (1),
lower to forward position (2), high
position (3), return to starting
position (4).

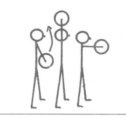

**E8   Straddle stance with ball
     in high position.**
Lower both arms to side shoulder
position, ball in left palm (1). Return
to starting position (2). Repeat to
other side.

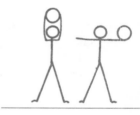

**E9   Straddle stance with ball
     in high position.**
Move the ball through a figure eight
pattern above the head. Repeat in
other direction.

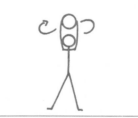

**E10 Straddle stance with ball in left
      shoulder position.**
Move the ball through a figure eight
pattern in the vertical plane. Note:
This may also be performed in the
horizontal plane.

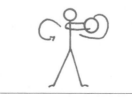

2.2 ARMS AND TRUNK

**E1 In a supported sitting position
with the feet up on the ball.**
Raise the hips to the horizontal
position (1). Return to the starting
position (2).

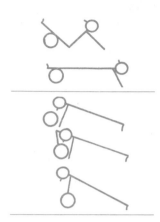

**E2 In a supported prone position
behind the ball.**
Take a left, then a right hand support
on the ball (1-2). Return to the
starting position (3-4).

**E3 In a supported sitting position
with the feet (slightly apart) up on
the ball.**
Raise the hips and turn left to a side
supported position (1). Return to the
starting position (2). Repeat turning
to the other side.

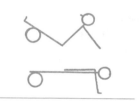

**E4 In a push-up position with the feet
supported on the ball.**
Lower chest to floor (1), return to
starting position (2).

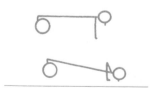

**E5 In a supported prone position
behind the ball with legs straddled.**
Perform a dynamic push-up to hands
supported on ball (1). Return to start
(2). Repeat.

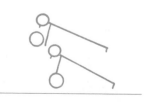

**E6 In a supported squat position
with hands on the ball.**
Reach forward with the ball (1), hop
legs forward to starting position (2).
Repeat continuously with rhythm.

**E7 Exactly as exercise E6, except that
the ball is held between the ankles.**

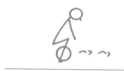

**E8 In a supported prone position,
with hands on the ball and legs
straddled.**
Move forward by rolling the ball with
alternating hand movements.

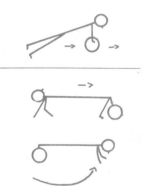

**E9 In a supported supine position
with feet on the ball (knees bent).**
Move forward by rolling the ball
with alternating leg movements.

**E10 In a supported prone position
(with feet on the ball).**
Walk with hands in a circle to the left
around the ball. Repeat to the other
side. (This exercise may be done with
the hands supported on the ball as
well.)

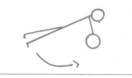

2.3 ABANDOMINALS I

E1 **Supine position, ball in high position.**
On ground, raise ball to front shoulder position and raise legs to touch ball (1), lower to starting position (2).

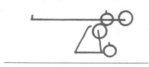

E2 **Supported sitting position, with ball held between ankles, knees bent.**
Extend knees to high diagonal position (1) and lower to starting position (2).

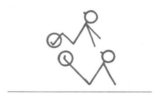

E3 **Supported sitting position, with ball held between the ankles, legs straight.**
Raise legs to high diagonal position (1) and lower to starting position (2).

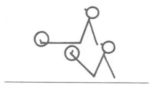

E4 **Basic supine position with ball held between the ankles.**
Raise the legs to vertical position (1), lower to starting position (2).

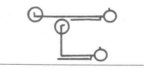

E5 **Supported sitting position with ball held between the ankles.**
Move the ball in an arc to the left (1). Return to starting position (2). Repeat to right side.

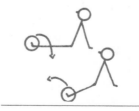

E6 **Supine position with legs in vertical position, ball between ankles.**
Bend at knees and lower ball to ground by rolling hips to the left (1). Return to the starting position (2). Repeat to right side.

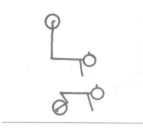

E7 **Supine position, arms in high position with the ball held between the ankles.**
Raise the legs and move the ball to a position on the ground over the head (1). Return to starting position (2).

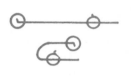

E8 **In pairs. "A" in supine position with legs in vertical position and arms behind head, ball held with ankles.**
"B" in supported squat position holding "A"'s arms on ground. "A" lowers ball to left side touching ground (1). Return to starting position (2). Repeat to opposite side. Change positions and repeat.

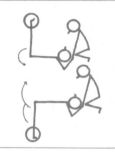

E9 **Basic supine position with ball in high position.**
Raise arms and legs to V-sit (1). Return to the starting position (2).

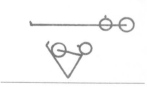

E10 **In pairs. "A" in basic supine position with ball held by ankles and arms behind the head.**
"B" in supported squat position holding "A" s arms on ground. "A" raises legs and hips (1). Return to starting position (2). Change positions and repeat.

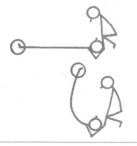

2.4 ABDOMINALS II

E1 Basic siting position with ball held in front of chest.
Lower to supine position (1),.return to starting position (2).

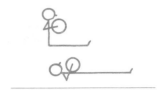

E2 In forearm supported sitting position with ball held between the ankles.
Raise the legs to 45° (1). Lower to starting position (2).

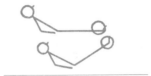

E3 In straddle supine position with ball on chest.
Sit-up to seated position while raising ball to high position (1). Return to starting position (2).

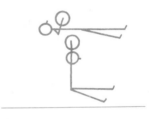

E4 In straddle sitting position with ball in forward position.
Roll back and raise ball to high position on the floor while bringing legs over to feet on ball (1). Return to starting position (2).

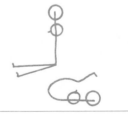

E5 In bent knee sitting position with ball behind neck.
Partner firmly holding the ankles. Lower to supine position (1) and return to starting position (2).Change positions and repeat.

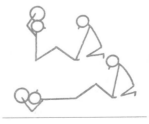

E6 **In bent knee supine position
with ball on top of head.**
Slowly curl up (1) and return to
starting position (2).

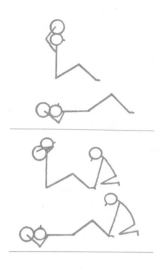

E7 **In bent knee position with ball held
in high position.**
Slowly curl up (1) and return to
starting position (2).

E8 **As in exercise E5, with ball held
at the chest.**
Lower to supine position while
raising the ball to the high position
(1), return to starting position (2).

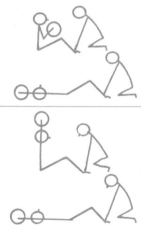

E9 **As in exercise E5, with ball held in
high position throughout the
exercise.**

E10 **As in exercise E5, with ball behind
the neck.**
With flat back (and tilted pelvis)
lower back to 45° and hold (1).
Return to starting position (2).
Note: This exercise may be done with the
same progressions as seen in the previous
exercises by alternating the ball position to
create greater resistance.

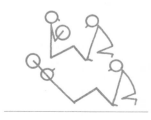

2.5 BACK EXERCISES

E1 Kneeling behind the ball with arms in high position.
With a flat back, bend forward to hands supported on ball. Trunk bouncing 3 times (1-3), return to starting position (4).

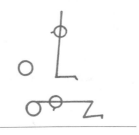

E2 Straddle stance with the ball behind the neck.
With a flat back, bend forward (1). Return to starting position (2).

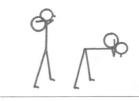

E3 Kneeling behind the ball with the arms in side shoulder position.
With a flat back, bend forward to hands supported on the ball and left leg extended sideways. Trunk bouncing 3 times (1-3), return to starting position (4). Repeat to other side.

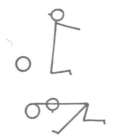

E4 Straddle stance with ball on top of head.
With a flat back, bend forward and bounce gently 3 times (1-3), return to starting position (4).

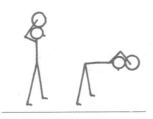

E5 Reclining in a straddle position, with neck supported on the ball, hands on the hips.
Raise the hips (1), lower to starting position (2).

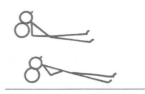

**E6   Bent over straddle stance with flat
      back and ball held on floor beneath
      the shoulders (forward position).**
Raise ball to horizontal (high
position) and lower to starting
position (2).

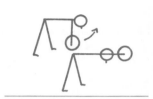

**E7   Basic erect stance with ball
      in deep position.**
With a flat back and straight left leg,
slowly lower ball to floor as left leg is
raised (to arabesque) (1). Slowly
return to starting position (2). Repeat
to other side.

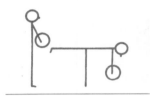

**E8   Basic erect stance with ball
      in high position.**
Lower ball to top of head while
moving slowly to arabesque position
- left leg raised (1). Slowly return to
starting position (2). Repeat to other
side.

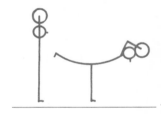

**E9   Straddle stance with ball held
      in front of chest.**
With a flat back, bend the trunk
forward while extending the arms and
ball to high position (1). Return to
starting position (2).

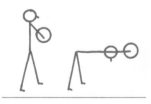

**E10 Basic erect stance with ball
      in high position.**
This exercise is exactly as E8, except
that the ball is maintained in the *high
position.*

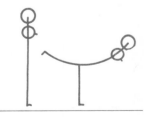

2.6 BACK EXERCISES FROM A LYING POSITION

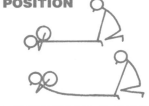

**E1 Lying in prone position with ball held
behind the neck.**
Partner holding the ankles.
Slowly curl the upper trunk (1). Return to
starting position (2).

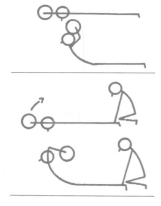

**E2 In prone position with the ball held
in the high position.**
Raise the legs and curl the upper
trunk backwards while lowering ball
to top of head.

**E3 In prone position with ball held in
the high position.**
Partner firmly holding the ankles.
Curl the upper trunk backwards and
raises from the floor while lowering
ball to behind neck (1). Return to
starting position (2).

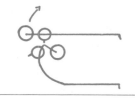

**E4 As exercise E3 without assistance
of partner.**

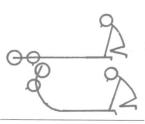

**E5 As in exercise E3, except that the
ball is held in high position.**

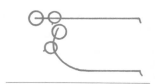

E6 As in exercise E5 without assistance of partner.

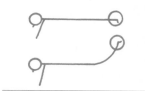

E7 In prone position with arms in side shoulder position and ball held between the ankles.
Raise the legs (1) and lower to starting position (2).

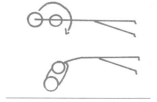

E8 In straddle position with ball held in high position.
Raise ball through an arc to the left (1).
Return to starting position through the same arc (2).
Repeat to other side.

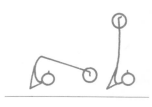

E9 In supported shoulder stance with the ball held between the ankles.
Lower legs behind head until ball touches the floor (1). Return to starting position (2).

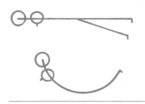

E10 In straddle prone position with ball held in high position.
Raise legs and bring them together while curling the upper trunk backwards and lifting ball high (1).
Return to starting position (2).

2.7 LEGS AND HIPS

E1 **In a supported sitting position with ball held between the ankles.**
Bend the knees to the chest (1), extend to starting position (2).

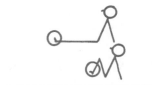

E2 **Lying in a prone position with arms in side shoulder position, ball held between the ankles.**
Bend the knees to raise the ball to a vertical position (1), lower to starting position (2).

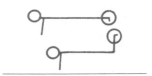

E3 **Standing with the ball held between the knees.**
Hop forwards and backwards.

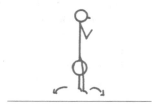

E4 **Standing with the ball held between the ankles.**
Hop forwards and backwards.

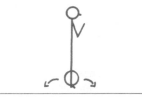

E5 **Basic erect stance with ball in high position.**
Lower to kneeling position with single leg support and lower ball to forward position (1). Return to starting position (2). Repeat using other leg to lower.

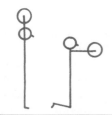

E6 **Basic erect stance with ball in high position.**
Lower ball to the floor to a supported lunge position with left leg extended (1). Return to starting position (2). Repeat to other side.

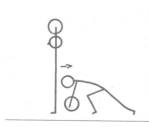

E7 **Basic erect stance with ball in high position.**
Lower ball to floor to a supported squat position with left leg extended laterally (1). Return to starting position (2).

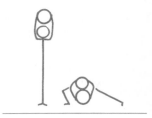

E8 **Basic erect stance with the ball held behind the neck.**
Step forward to left lunge position and bounce 3 times to touch ball to floor (1-3). Return to starting position (4). Repeat to other side.

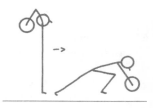

E9 **In a squat stance with ball on top of head.**
Extend the left leg laterally (1), return to starting position (2). Repeat to other side.

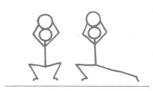

E10 **Kneeling with the ball in high position.**
Sit to the floor to the left (1), return to starting position (2). Repeat to other side.

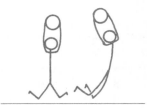

2.8 MORE DEMANDING LEG EXERCISES

E1 **In supported squat position
with hands on the ball.**
Step with left leg to a long lunge and raise
ball to high position (1). Return to starting
position (2). Repeat to other side.

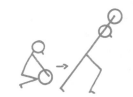

E2 **In supported squat position with
hands on the ball.**
Step with the left leg to a side lunge
position and raise the ball to the high
position and bounce 3 times (1-3).
Return to starting position (4). Repeat
to other side.

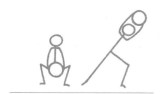

E3 **Basic erect stance with the ball held
in front of the chest.**
Lower to squat (1). Hold. Rise to 1/2
squat (2). Hold. Rise to 1/4 squat (3).
Hold. Return to starting position (4).

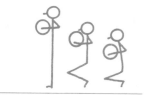

E4 **In squat position with the ball
on the chest.**
Extend left leg laterally and raise ball
to high position (1). Return to starting
position (2). Repeat to opposite side.

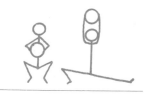

E5 **In squat position with the ball
on the chest.**
Bounce 3 times (1-3) and leap into
the air extending ball to forward
position (4).

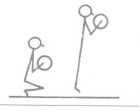

E6 **Erect stance with ball held
on the chest.**
Lower to squat position and hop
forwards 3 times (1-3). Return to
starting position (4).

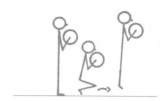

E7 **Squat with the ball behind
the neck.**
Hop forwards, 4 times (1-4) and then
hop back 4 times (5-8).

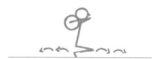

E8 **Squat position with ball
in deep position.**
Long hop forwards with body
extension, swing back to forward
position - land in starting position.
Repeat.

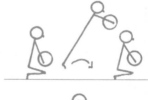

E9 **Squat position with ball
in deep position.**
Leap to high body extension with
straddled legs and swing ball to high
position - land in the starting position.

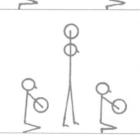

E10 **In straddle stance with bent knees
and ball held in right side shoulder
position.**
Leap to a high position and complete
a 360° turn moving ball to left side
shoulder position.

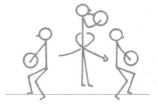

2.9 GENERAL EXERCISES

E1 **Wide straddle stance with ball on top of head.**
With deep left knee bend, lean to the left and raise the ball to the high position (1). Return to starting position (2). Repeat to opposite side.

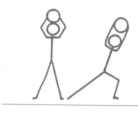

E2 **Basic erect stance with ball behind the neck.**
Step forward to a left lunge position and in front lean raise the ball to the high position (1). Return to starting position (2). Repeat to opposite side.

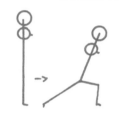

E3 **In pairs. With a strong grasp on the ball, partners attempt to wrestle it away from each other.**
This exercise may be done in a kneeling or sitting position as well.

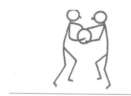

E4 **In supine lying position with the ball held between the ankles.**
Roll backwards to place the ball on the floor over head (1). Leaving the ball, lower the legs to starting position (2).
Sit up with the ball in the high position and place it between the ankles (3). Leaving the ball, return to starting position (4).

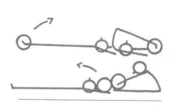

E5 **Basic sitting position with the ball in high position.**
Do a complete roll to the left to the supine position (1), to prone (2), to supine (3). Sit up to starting position (4). Repeat to the other side.

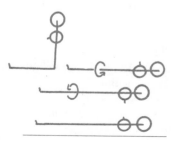

E6 In supine lying position with ball held in high position.

Do a complete roll to the left through the prone position to the supine again (1). Sit to a V-sit and touch ball with toes (2). Lower to starting position (3). Repeat to other side.

E7 Erect stance with ball in forward position.

Through sitting lower to supine position and return to starting position the same way. Maintain constant ball position throughout.

E8 Erect stance with ball in high position.

Through kneeling, side sitting and side lying to prone position. Return to starting position the same way. Maintain constant ball position throughout.

E9 In pairs. Partners stand back to back and hold a medicine ball between their backs.

Walk around to left and then to right and finally sit down and stand up without losing the ball. Do not use hands.

E10 In pairs. Partners stand with the ball held between their foreheads.

Walk around to left and to right and then lower to support kneeling position and stand up.

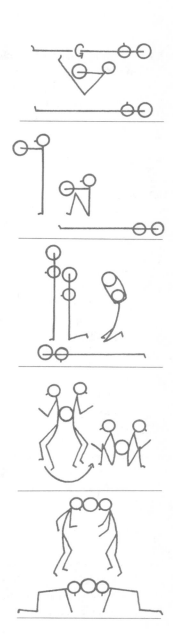

3.1 UNDERHAND THROWS

**E1 Straddle stance with ball
in deep position.**
"A" with back flat bends forward and
rolls the ball to "B". "B" bends
forward to receive ball and rolls it
back. Both return to erect position
between throws.

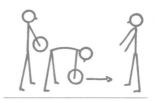

**E2 Seated straddle with ball
in deep position.**
"A" rolls ball to "B" who rolls it
back.

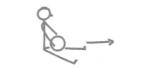

**E3 Straddle stance with ball
in deep position.**
"A" with back flat bends forward and
throws the ball to "B", returning to
erect position. "B" receives ball and
bends forward to set up throw to "A".

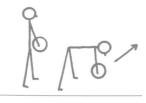

**E4 Straddle stance with ball
in high position.**
"A" with back flat swings ball down
between legs and throws it to "B",
returning to erect position. "B"
receives ball in high position and
repeats motion.

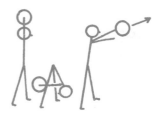

**E5 Basic kneeling position
with ball in deep position.**
"A" throws underhand to "B" who
returns the ball in the same manner.

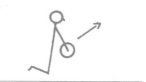

**E6   Seated straddle position with ball
      in deep position.**
"A" throws underhand to "B" who
returns the ball in the same manner.

**E7   Basic erect stance with ball
      in deep position.**
"A" with back flat bends forward and
throws ball to "B", returning to erect
position. "B" receives ball and returns
it in the same manner.

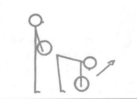

**E8   "A" in basic erect stance with ball
      in deep position. "B" in deep squat.**
"A" throws underhand to "B" who
rises to receive ball. "A" squats after
throw. Repeat action as "B" returns
throw.

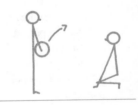

**E9   "A" in basic erect stance with ball
      in deep position. "B" in basic
      kneeling position.**
"A" throws underhand to "B" who
rises to receive ball. "A" drops to
kneeling position. Repeat action as
"B" returns throw.

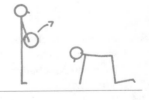

**E10 "A" in basic erect position with ball
      in deep position. "B" in supported
      prone position.**
"A" throws underhand to "B" who
rises to receive ball. "A" drops to
kneeling position. Repeat action as
"B" returns throw.

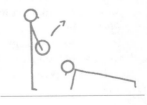

3.2 PUSH FORWARD THROWS

**E1 Basic erect stance with ball
in deep position.**
"A" steps forward with left foot and
brings ball to chest position to push
ball to "B". "B" returns throw.

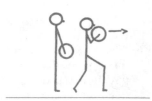

**E2 Straddle stance with ball
in chest position.**
Push the ball forward (1). Return to
original position (2).

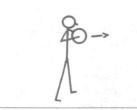

**E3 Basic straddle stance with ball in
putting position on right shoulder
supported by hand.**
Push ball to partner who receives it
in front shoulder position. Take ball
to right shoulder with trunk twist
and return it. Repeat alternating
pushing arm.

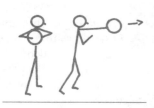

**E4 Seated straddle position
with ball at chest.**
Push and pass ball to partner
with rhythm.

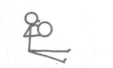

**E5 Seated straddle position with ball
in putting position on right
shoulder supported by left hand.**
Push ball to partner who receives it in
front shoulder position. Take ball to
right shoulder with trunk twist and
return it. Repeat alternating pushing
arm.

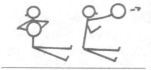

E6   Straddle stance with ball at chest. "A" has back to "B".
With knee bounce "A" throws ball over head to "B". "B" turns to throw and "A" turns to receive. Repeat rhythmically.

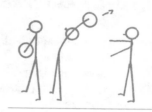

E7   Basic erect stance with ball at chest.
Lower to squat and bounce twice. On third bounce drive up and push ball to partner. Partner receives standing and repeats.

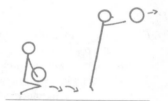

E8   Supine position with ball at chest.
Sit up and push ball to partner who is seated in a straddle position. Partner lays back, sits up and repeats action.

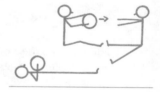

E9   Squat position with ball at chest.
With rhythmic knee bouncing pass ball vigorously back and forth between partners.

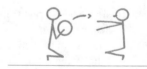

E10 Straddle prone position with ball at forehead.
Raise trunk and push ball to partner. Continue throws rhythmically.

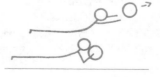

3.3 OVERHEAD THROWS

E1 **Basic erect stance with ball
in deep position.**
Swing ball to high position stepping
forward with left foot, and throw
overhand to partner.

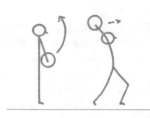

E2 **Basic erect stance with ball
in deep position.**
Swing ball to behind neck stepping
forward with left foot, and throw
overhand to partner.

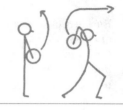

E3 **Straddle with ball in deep position.**
Swing ball to high position and
throw overhand to partner.

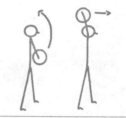

E4 **Basic kneeling position with ball
in deep position.**
Swing ball to behind neck position
and throw overhand to partner.

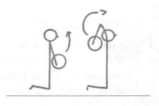

E5 **Kneeling lunge position with
left leg forward and ball in
high position.**
Throw rhythmically back and forth
lowering ball to behind neck each
time.

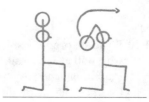

E6   **Seated, ball in deep position.**
Swing to behind neck and throw
to partner.

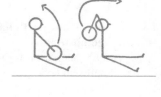

E7   **Basic erect stance with ball
in deep position.**
Lower to deep squat stance and
swing ball to high position and
throw overhand to partner.

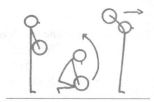

E8   **Basic erect stance with ball
in deep position.**
Step forward and swing ball to
deep throwing position supported
with other hand, throw to partner.
Alternate throwing arm.

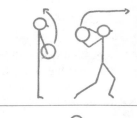

E9   **Seated with ball in high position.**
Roll back and bring feet over your
head (1). Return to original position
and throw ball to partner (2).

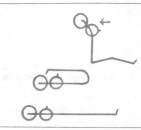

E10 **Prone position with ball
in high position.**
As trunk is raised, ball is taken to
behind neck and thrown overhand
to partner.

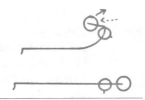

3.4 BACKWARD UNDERHAND THROWS

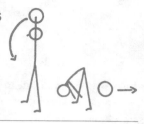

E1   **Straddle stance with ball
in high position.**
With flat back bend forward and roll
ball between legs to partner.

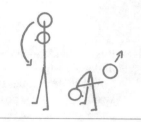

E2   **Straddle stance with ball
in high position.**
With flat back bend forward and
throw the ball between legs to
partner.

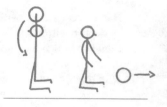

E3   **Kneeling with ball in high position.**
Swing ball down to left side and roll
to partner. Alternate sides
rhythmically.

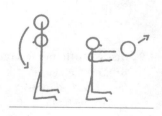

E4   **Kneeling with ball in high position.**
Swing ball down to left side and
throw to partner. Alternate sides
rhythmically.

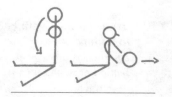

E5   **Seated straddle position
with ball in high position.**
Swing ball down to left side and
roll to partner. Alternate sides
rhythmically.

E6 Seated straddle position with ball in high position.
Swing ball down to left side and throw to partner. Alternate sides rhythmically.

E7 Basic erect stance with ball in high position.
Swing ball down to left side and lower to deep squat to roll ball to partner.

E8 Basic erect stance with ball in high position.
Swing ball down to the left side and lower to deep squat to throw ball to partner.

E9 Basic erect stance with ball in high position.
Swing ball down to the left side and throw to partner. Repeat to the other side.

E10 Basic erect stance with ball in high position.
Jump to straddle position as ball is swung down and thrown between legs to partner.

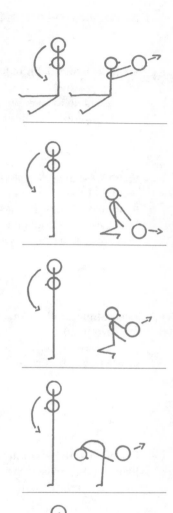

3.5 BACKWARD OVERHEAD THROWS

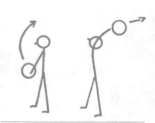

E1 **Straddle stance with ball
in deep position.**
Swing ball up to be thrown overhead
and backwards to partner.

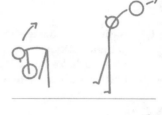

E2 **Straddle stance with slight knee
bend and flat-backed forward
bend, ball in forward position.**
Swing trunk and ball up to be thrown
overhead and backwards to partner.

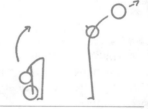

E3 **Erect stance and flat-backed
forward bend.**
Swing trunk and ball up to be thrown
overhead and backwards to partner.

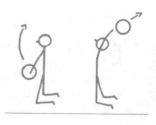

E4 **Kneeling with ball in deep position.**
Swing ball up to be thrown overhead
and backwards to partner.

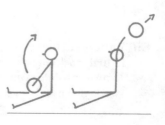

E5 **Seated straddle position
with ball in deep position.**
Swing ball up to be thrown overhead
and backwards to partner.

E6 **Seated straddle position with
ball extended far forward.**
Swing ball up to be thrown overhead
and backwards to partner.

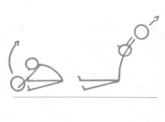

E7 **Deep squat position with ball
in deep position.**
Stand up and swing ball to be thrown
overhead and backwards to partner.

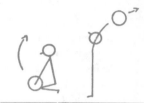

E8 **Straddle stance with slight knee
bend and flat-backed forward
bend, ball in forward position.**
Stand up and swing the ball to the left
side to partner. Alternate sides.

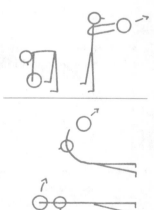

E9 **Straddle prone position
with ball in high position.**
Raise trunk and swing ball backwards
and overhead to partner.

E10 **Straddle prone position
with ball in high position.**
Raise trunk and swing ball backwards
over the left shoulder. Alternate sides.

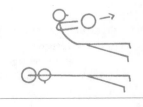

3.6 SWINGING THROWS

**E1   Straddle stance with ball
in deep position.**
Swing ball to right and back down
again with knee bounce to roll it to
partner who receives it and returns it
rhythmically.

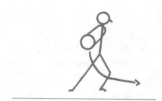

**E2   Straddle stance with ball
in deep position.**
Swing ball to right and back down
again with knee bounce to throw it at
partner who receives it and returns it
rhythmically.

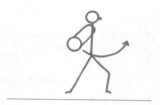

**E3   Straddle stance with ball in right-
side shoulder position.**
Swing ball across flatly to be thrown
to partner.

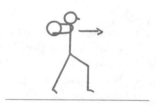

**E4   Basic erect stance with ball
in back deep position.**
Step forward with left leg and throw
ball overhead to partner.

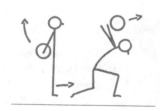

**E5   Straddle stance with ball
in deep position.**
Swing ball to the right and up to
be thrown over the head to partner
on left.

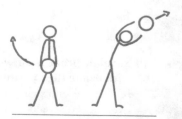

**E6   Straddle stance with ball
       in deep position.**
Lower to deep squat and swing ball to
side shoulder position on right.
Return to stand and swing ball across
to throw to partner on left.

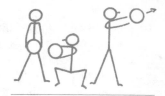

**E7   Straddle stance with ball
       in deep position.**
Swing back on left side to throw it
flatly forward to partner. Alternate
sides.

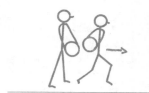

**E8   Straddle stance with knees flexed
       and ball in side shoulder position
       with trunk twist.**
(Supported throwing position.)
Throw ball with one hand to partner.
Alternate sides.

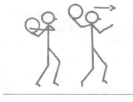

**E9   Basic erect stance with ball held
       between the ankles.**
With a jump, throw ball to partner.

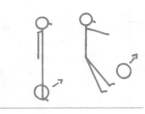

**E10 Seated position with ball
       between the ankles.**
Rock back to supported shoulder
stance and throw ball to partner.

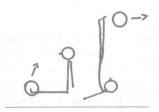

3.7 USING TWO BALLS

**E1 "A" and "B" in straddle stance
face to face.**
"A" from deep position - ball is rolled
along the floor to "B". "B" from chest
position - ball is thrown flatly to "A".

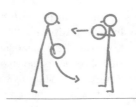

**E2 "A" and "B" in straddle stance
face to face.**
"A" from deep position - ball is rolled
along the floor to "B". "B" from high
position - ball is thrown flatly to "A".

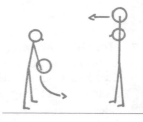

**E3 "A" and "B" in straddle stance
side by side.**
"A" from deep position - ball is
rolled along the floor to "B". "B"
from high position - ball is thrown
laterally to "A".

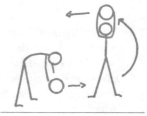

**E4 "A" and "B" in straddle stance
facing in same direction.**
"A" from deep position - ball is
rolled along the floor between "B"'s
legs. "B" from high position - ball is
thrown backward to "A".

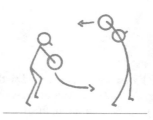

**E5 "A" and "B" in straddle stance,
knees flexed, face to face.**
"A" from deep position - ball is
thrown flatly to "B". "B" from chest
position - ball is thrown flatly to "A".

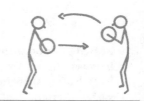

E6 **"A" and "B" in straddle stance, knees flexed, face to face.**
"A" from deep position - ball is thrown flatly to "B". "B" from high position - ball is thrown flatly to "A".

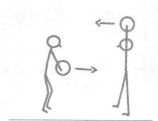

E7 **"A" and "B" in seated straddle position face to face.**
"A" from chest position - ball is thrown flatly across to "B". "B" from chest position - ball is thrown higher to "A".

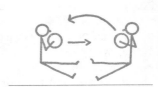

E8 **"A" and "B" in prone position face to face.**
"A" pushes ball along floor to "B". "B" - from elevated position ball is thrown to "A".

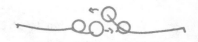

E9 **"A" and "B" facing in same direction.**
"A" from prone position, trunk is raised and ball is thrown overhead and backwards to "B". "B" from flat-backed, bent over straddle stance, ball is rolled to side of "A".

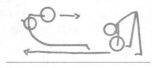

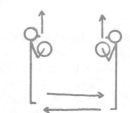

E10 **"A" and "B" face to face, basic erect stance, ball at chest.**
"A" and "B" throw ball into air and run to catch partner's ball. Repeat.

3.8 INDIVIDUAL EXERCISES

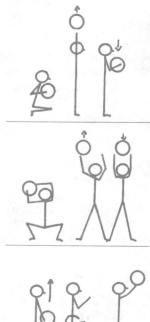

E1 **Deep squat with ball at chest.**
Rise to erect stance and drive ball
into the air. Catch it and lower to
deep squat. Repeat rhythmically.

E2 **Deep squat with ball supported
on shoulder.**
Jump to straddle stance and drive ball
up with one hand. Catch it above
head, lower to the shoulder and return
to deep squat. Repeat rhythmically.

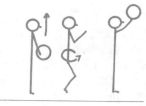

E3 **Basic erect stance with ball
in deep position.**
Throw ball into the air and hop
through a 360° turn. Catch ball,
lower it, and repeat.

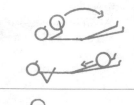

E4 **Straddle supine position with legs
raised and ball at chest.**
Throw ball to be caught by ankles
and allowed to roll down legs to
hands. Repeat rhythmically.

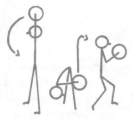

E5 **Straddle stance with ball
in high position.**
With flat back bend forward and
swing ball down to be thrown up
between legs. Execute a quick jump
turn to catch ball and repeat.

**E6   Erect stance with ball
between ankles.**
Throw ball up behind the back to left
side and catch it. Drop ball to floor
and repeat to other side.

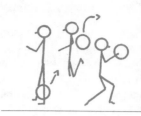

**E7   Basic erect stance with ball
in deep position.**
Throw ball up and catch it behind in
deep position. Throw it up and to
front and continue.

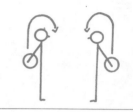

**E8   Basic erect stance with ball
in deep position.**
Throw ball up and lower to supported
deep squat position. Rise up to catch
ball and repeat.

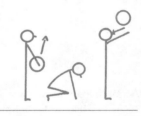

**E9   Straddle stance with ball
in high position.**
With flat back bend forward and
swing ball down to be thrown up
between legs and over head and
caught in front. Repeat.

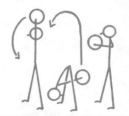

**E10 Basic erect stance
with ball between ankles.**
Throw the ball up behind the back
and over the shoulder to be caught
in front. Repeat.

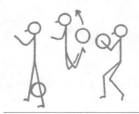

4.1 COMPETITIONS

Athletes standing on starting line (or depending on the assignment - kneeling, sitting, lying, etc.) with one or more balls with 1.5 - 2 metres between them. At the starting signal the competitors run, hop, bounce, etc. to the finish line. The distance between the start and finish line will vary from 10 to 30 metres depending upon the age and ability level of the participants, the difficulty of the task (hopping as opposed to running), etc.

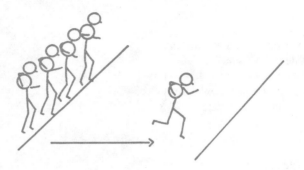

Variations

A. Running with 1, 2, or 3, medicine balls held in the hands. May also be done with backwards running.

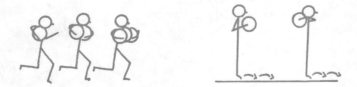

B. Hopping with both legs with ball on chest or on neck. May also be done with backwards hopping.

C. Hopping on single leg with one or two balls held in the hands.

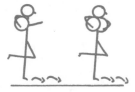 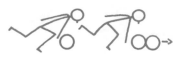

D. Running while rolling one or two balls along the ground.

E. Walking on the knees with one or two balls in the hands. May also be done while rolling the balls as in D.

 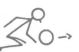   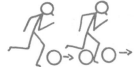

F. Dribbling the ball with the feet (as in soccer) using one or two balls.

G. In all fours position with ball held in the hands or between the ankles hopping forwards.

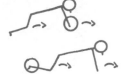
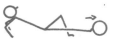

H. In crab walk position (hands over feet face up) dribbling the ball with the feet.

I. On hands and knees dribbling the ball with head.

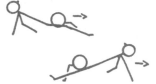

J. In crab walk position with the ball held in the lap move either (i) forward or (ii) backwards.

4.2 RELAYS

Arrange teams of equal numbers (and at roughly equal ability) behind the
starting line in rows behind a leader. Space the teams 2-3 metres apart. In front
of each team, 10 to 30 metres away, place an adequate marker on the ground.
Competitors may pass around it to the left or to the right. The distance to the
marker will depend upon all the usual variables of age, fitness, etc. At the
starting signal the first athlete will run, hop, etc. to the marker passing around
it left or right and return to his/her team. After exchanging the ball (or balls) to
the next athlete in line s/he goes to the end of the row. The race goes on until
all members have completed the circuit once or more. Winners any be
determined by the team that crosses the starting line first upon completion, or
by a whole variety of fun assignments such as seated, seated cross-legged,
kneeling, etc. and/or with various hand positions such as on top of the head.
This can add a true element of "mental challenge" and fun.

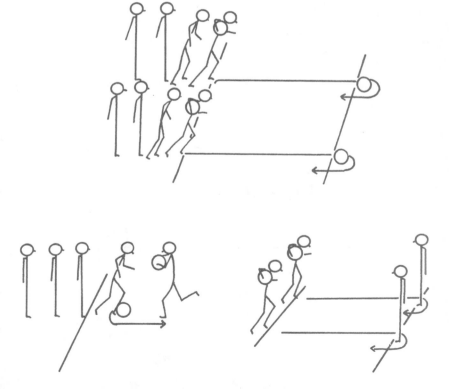

4.3 THROWING COMPETITIONS

Arrange individuals to form teams with lines beside each other (spaced 4-8 metres apart) with 3-4 metres between each team. On each team the member on the right end of the line has one medicine ball. At the starting signal the ball is thrown sideways successively along the line to the end and then back to the leader.

As with all competitions the ball may go one or more times up and down the line; the athletes may be standing, kneeling, seated, and the variations of throwing the ball are unlimited: underhand, overhand, etc.

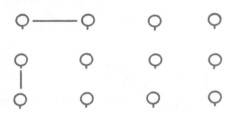

4.4 BALL PASSING RELAYS

Arrange teams in rows, team members spaced about 1 metre apart and 2-3 metres separating each team. Each athlete is standing with legs straddled and the leader has a medicine ball.

At the starting signal the leader passes the ball backwards over his/her head to the second athlete who passes it along in the same fashion. The last athlete in the row runs with the ball on the left of the row to the front and repeats the process. The competition continues until the original leader is at the front of the row again.

The relay can also be done by passing the ball between the legs.

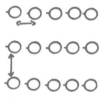

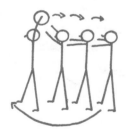

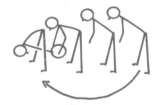

Variations:

A. The team members alternate passing the ball over the head and between the legs.

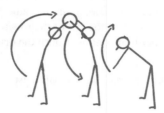

B. The last team member, instead of running forward, may crawl forward between the straddled legs with the ball.

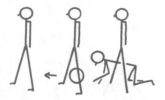   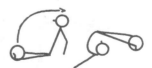

C. The team members, about 2 metres apart, and the ball held between the ankles pass the ball back by rolling the legs up over the head and passing the ball in this fashion.

4.5 BALL CHASING GAMES

A. Work with an even number of athletes, join hands in a circle, release hands and step two strides backwards. Assign numbers around the circle by 2's (1-2; 1-2). The 1's are a team, the 2's are the other team. At one point on the circle a "1" has the ball and directly across a "2" has a ball. At the starting signal the balls are passed to the left to the other members of the team. If a team catches the other a point is awarded.

The variations are almost limitless related to the method of throwing (underhand, overhand, putting, etc.) and the posture of the athlete (standing, sitting, kneeling). Pass the ball in both directions.

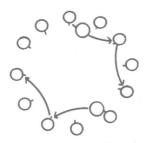
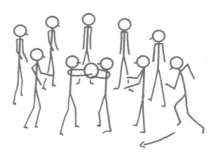

B. The difference in this game is that an athlete chases the ball and there are no teams. An athlete starts across the circle from the ball and at the signal begins to run in the direction that the ball is being passed. Each person must handle the ball. When the runner touches the ball s/he assumes the position of the passer and the passer becomes the runner. Again, the method of passing and the directions of the throw may be changed.

i) A variation is that passes are made under the raised leg in a seated position.

ii) A second variation is rolling the ball between the legs in a straddle stance.

4.6. MULTIPLE BALL PASSING GAMES

Each athlete in the circle has a ball and at the signal passes it to the right (or left) and must quickly receive the ball being passed to him/her.

i) A variation is to pass in command — left, left, etc. and insert a change of direction occasionally.
ii) Wwalking in a circle (spaced 3-4 metres) on every eighth stride the ball is thrown up and caught again.
iii) As in ii) but the ball is thrown overhead backwards to be caught by the athlete following.
iv) All of the above variations done while jogging or running.

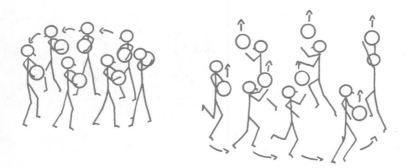

4.7 SPIDER OR CRAB SOCCER

Basically all the rules of soccer apply (on a small playing surface) but movement is only allowed in the back supported position.

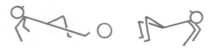

4.8 "FORCE OUT"

With 3-10 athletes on each team facing each other, a ball is thrown back and forth, the object being to force the opposing team back out of its court across the base line. A ball that is caught permits three strides before returning it, a ball that hits the floor must be thrown from that spot.

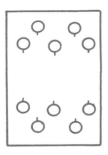

4.9 "STRING BALL" (VOLLEYBALL RULES THROWING A MEDICINE BALL)

Court size will depend upon the number of athletes per team. A string is placed across the centre court 2-2.5 metres high. There is a restraining line 2 metres on either side of the centre. The ball may not be thrown from inside this area and it is classed out of bounds as all the other out-of-court areas.

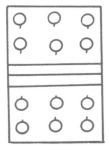

Notes

Notes

Notes

Notes

Notes